# 30 - DAY
# Flat Belly Guide

Diet and Exercise Secrets For Burning Belly
Fat Fast –
No Fluff, Just Facts!

by FlatBelly Queens

Published in Great Britain by:

FlatBelly Queens
345 Old Street
London
EC1V 9LE

© Copyright 2016 – Flatbelly Queens

ISBN-13: {978-1533320124}
ISBN-10: {1533320128}

# Table of Contents

# INTRODUCTION

Thank you for downloading the 30-Day Flat Belly Guide.

In the next chapters, we will help you develop awesome abs and get rid of belly fat in 30 days. It is not only intended to make you look better as you achieve your ideal body shape, but actually make you healthier. You see these gorgeous women with sexy abs on television, but how did they get them? Truth is, it's not really that hard to develop strong stomach muscles. You just need to know what to do and stick to it.

Love handles, jellyrolls, spare tires, and potbellies – we give it cute names and laugh it off. However, belly fat or visceral fat has been proven to be more dangerous to your health than you think. In fact, in a study presented at the European Society of Cardiology Congress, it was confirmed that having a lot of fat around your belly poses more of a health risk than being obese.

This study showed that cardiovascular deaths are 2.75 times higher for people who have normal body weight but big tummies, as compared to those with a normal waist-to-hip ratio. So, it's not just about having the right weight, but also where the fats are located.

The fat that accumulate in your lower body, giving you that "pear" shape is subcutaneous. But the fat in your midsection, in the abdominal area, is visceral. When you pinch your waist, what you feel is subcutaneous fat. Visceral fat lies deep within the abdomen, taking up the spaces between our internal organs.

Visceral fat has been positively linked to metabolic disorders, Type 2 Diabetes and cardiovascular disease on both sexes. In women, it has been associated with breast cancer and severe gallbladder diseases. Another reason why belly fat is so harmful, is that it is so near the portal vein. This vein carries the blood from the intestinal area to the liver where they affect the production of blood lipids. Substances that are released by visceral fat, such as free fatty acids, enter the portal vein, causing many negative conditions like high cholesterol, low HDL, high LDL and resistance to insulin.

Before, belly fat was accepted as normal when you reach middle age – all part of the aging process. Now, with our more sedentary lifestyles, this is a problem experienced by all ages. It happens more in women than men, unfortunately. The extra pounds that women accumulate due to lack of physical activity, somehow settle down in the midsection. This is not only caused by weight gain but a decrease in the levels of estrogen. Genes can also be blamed, as well as chronic stress.

The good news is that belly fat is easily remedied by diet and exercise, and the benefits are immediate. You'll look sexier and your blood pressure and cholesterol levels will go down. If you heed the suggestions in this book, in 30 days, you will see sculpted and toned abs instead of love handles! So, let's get started, shall we?

# CHAPTER 1

## 12 Easy Exercises that Build Awesome Abs

How can we develop awesome abs and get rid of belly fat once and for all? We have included the most effective exercises that can make you lose weight fast, tone your abdominal muscles and strengthen your core.

Choose from the selection of exercises and come up with a routine that you can do for 30 minutes daily – for the next 30 days. Combined with nutritious food, you can be sure that you'll be buff and healthy in no time. Women often result to crunches or sit-ups, targeting the area of the abdominal muscles, but this is not the way. A combination of cardiovascular exercises, targeted exercises and light weight training work best. Remember that when you lose weight, the body gets rid of belly fat first.

Here are some moves that can help you tone your abdominal muscles and strengthen your core.

# The Lunge Twist

This exercise targets the abs, buttocks, oblique and quads.

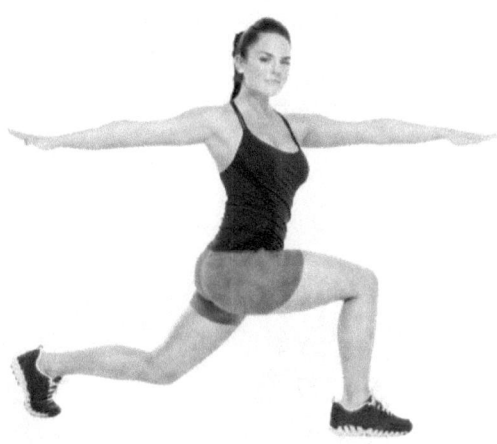

Stand with your feet a little apart, in line with your hips.
Knees should be a little bent and the hands on your sides
like in the above image.
Lunge forward with your right leg and twist your torso and
arms to the right.
Return to the center position.
Do 16 repetitions and alternate from a right lunge to the
left.

# Pilates 100

This Pilates move is easy and targets the stomach muscles and tones the thighs.

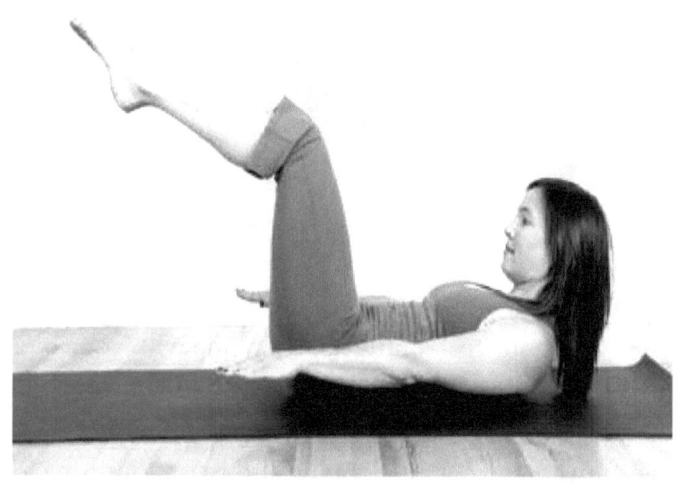

Lie down on your back with your arms by your sides. Keep your stomach and spine neutral and flat on the ground.
While contracting your abdominal muscles, bring both of your knees up.
Exhale then lift your head, shoulders and arms off the ground.

Straighten your legs as you lift, and pump your arms up and down while keeping it straight.
(As if your palms are pushing down on an invisible spring)
Inhale for 5 counts of arm pumps and exhale for another 5 and repeat up to 100 beats.

# Lunge with Dumbbells

This exercise targets the arms, abdominal muscles, quads and buttocks. Adding weights will intensify the effect of this lunge.

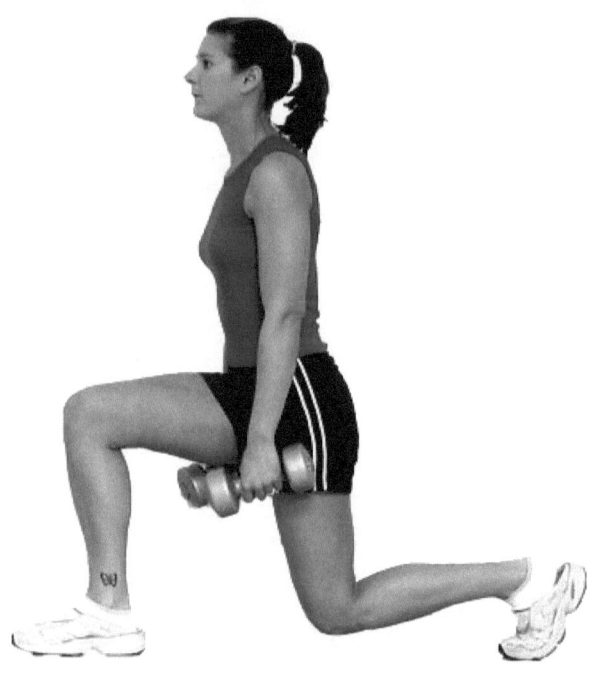

Article I.

Choose a weight that is not too light but not too heavy for you to lift over your head. (There should be some effort) Stand with your feet apart, in line with your hips.

Lunge forward with your left leg and bring your arms forward as you dip. Right in front of your toes. Forcefully push off with your left leg to return to the upright position. As you go up, lift both arms straight on top of your head. (Don't let go of that dumbbell!) Do 8 repetitions while switching sides.

# Interval Training

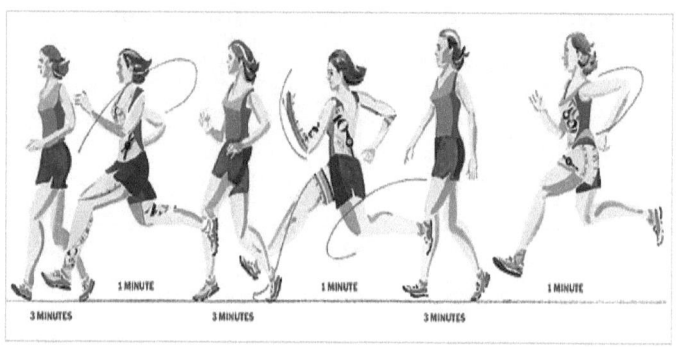

Cardio exercises are more effective and shows faster results when you apply interval training. What this means is, instead of a steady pace, you will do short bursts of high intensity workout and then return to the normal pace. You can apply this strategy while doing any type of cardio workout such as swimming, running, cycling, aerobics, etc. Incorporate interval training into your exercise and you will burn calories faster during the workout and even 24 to 48 hours after the routine.

Example: Run at a normal speed for 2 minutes, then run faster for 1 minute, then return to normal speed. Repeat this alternating pace for 20 minutes.

Do this for 3 times a week.

** Consult your doctor before doing high intensity exercises.

# Swimming

Swimming is a great way to burn fat around the belly since it gives you a total body workout. The trick is to keep your abdominals deliberately contracted as you paddle your feet.

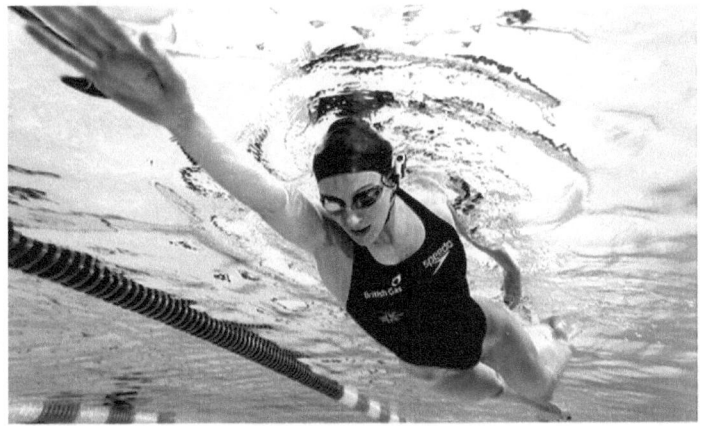

# The Superwoman

Strengthens not just the core, but also the lower back muscles.

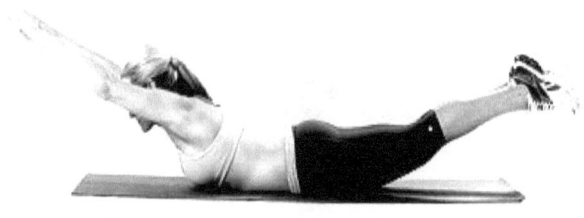

Lie face down on the ground, with your legs spread wider than your hips.
Extend your arms over your head, palms down and keep toes pointed.
(Like you're about to fly!)
Inhale as you raise your arms and legs as high as you can tolerate.
Hold the position for 5 seconds. Exhale as you slowly return to the first position.
Do 3 sets of 15 repetitions.

# Plank Pike Jacks with Sliding Discs

## Core and Strengthening Workout

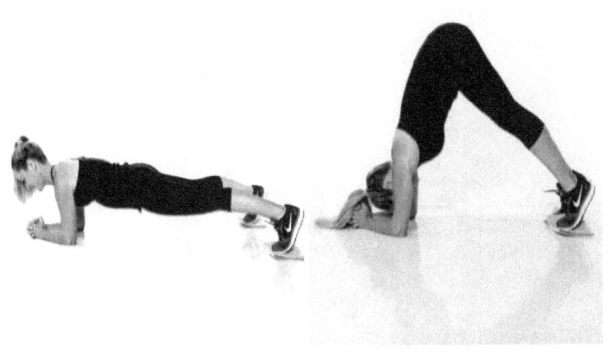

Start in a planking position, holding your body off the floor
using your elbows and toes.
(If you're at home, you can put anything that slides under
your toes – a rag, a small towel)
Use your core and tighten your abdominal muscles and slide
your feet towards your arms, pulling your glutes toward the
ceiling as you slide up.
Using your abdominal muscles, slide back down to plank
position.
Do 10 repetitions.

# Curtsy Lunge

This lunge is simple but works the buttocks, quadriceps, hamstrings and abdominal muscles.

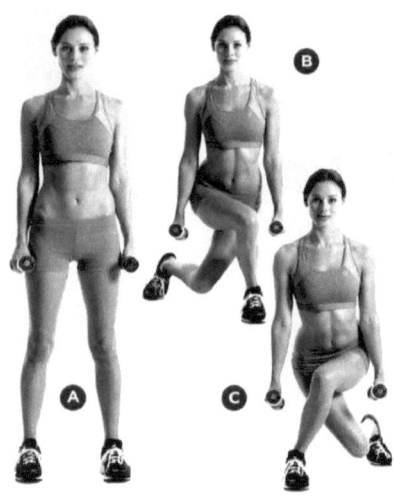

Hold light dumbbells and stand with your feet apart, hands on the sides.
Take a big step back diagonally with your left foot and cross it behind your right leg.
Bend knees in a curtsy while ensuring balance.
Return to your starting position.
Repeat with the other leg.
Do 3 sets of 15 repetitions.

# The Rolling Side Plank

A more difficult variation of the Plank, the side blank works your oblique and creates a strong core.

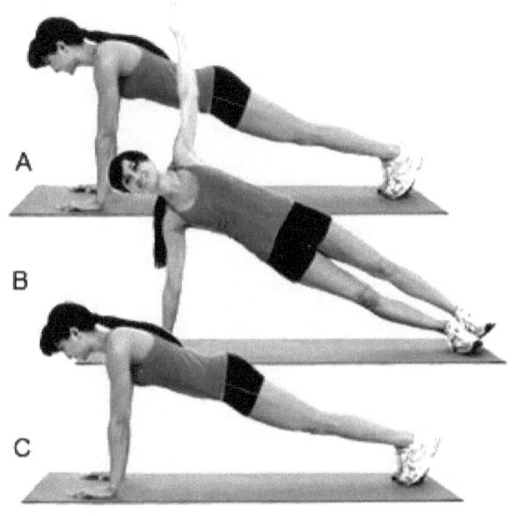

Start in the plank position with your arms and toes
supporting your body weight.
Shift your weight to your right arm and roll your body open
to the left side, extending your arm.
Hold the position for 30 to 60 seconds
Return to the plank position.
Repeat 15 times in 3 sets.

** You can adjust the level of difficulty depending on your capability. You can use your knees to support your weight as you turn on your sides. You can up the difficulty by lifting your other leg. There are many variations to the rolling side plank and you can play around with what you can do to further challenge your core.

# Single Leg Squats

Squats are the traditional way of working the abdominal muscles, but this single leg variation will give your workout that extra oomph.

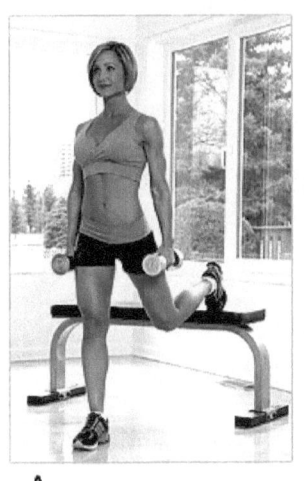 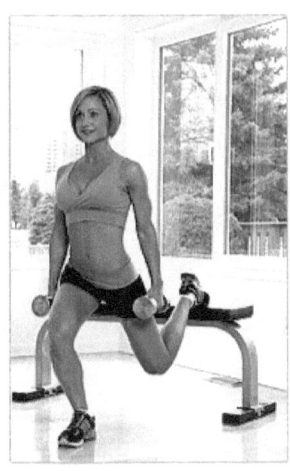

A.          B.

Stand on your right leg, left knee bent and foot lifted off the ground.
(You can use a chair or anything you can rest your foot on)
Hold the dumbbells on your sides.
Bend your right knee and squat on one foot, back foot supporting your balance.
Return to starting position and repeat with the other leg.
Do 3 sets of 10 repetitions.

# Single Leg Bridge

This exercise tones your back, lifts your buttocks, tones the thighs and sculpts your abdominal muscles. As you lift your legs, the abs work harder to stabilize your body.

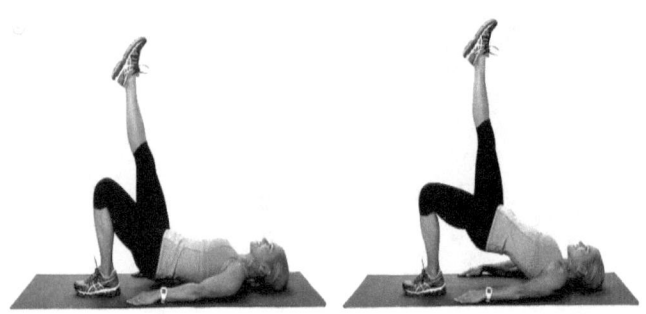

Lie flat on your back with both legs bent and feet flat on the ground or with feet flexed with only the heels touching the floor.

Your arms should be on your sides with palms down.
Stretch your right leg towards the ceiling, keeping it straight.
Tighten your abdominal muscles, press down with your left foot, and lift your hips as high as you can go.
Hold the position for 30 seconds.
Lower your hips to the ground.
Do 3 sets of 15 repetitions, alternating on each leg.

# Side Kick

Martial arts offer exercises that can seriously tone your body. The Side Kick may look like an easy exercise to do, but it's an abdominal toner. The oblique and abdominal muscles work hard to balance your body as you do your side kicks.

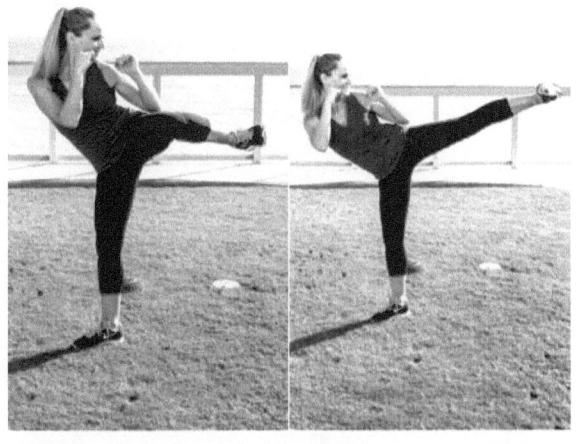

Stand with your arms bent, hands in fists under your chin. Shift your weight to your right foot, bend the right leg slightly and extend your left leg to the sides.

(Put some force to your kick, as if you're pushing something heavy with your extended leg)
Return to starting position.
Repeat this 15 times on the same leg and then switch to the other leg.
Do 3 sets.

# CHAPTER 2

## Belly-Fat Busting Recipes

Losing weight by eating the right foods and avoiding the wrong ones will help you in your goal of toning your abs and getting rid of unhealthy belly fat. Exercise alone won't work. Try the suggested recipes in this chapter and combine it with your daily exercise. If you take in more calories than you burn, it will be difficult to maintain a normal body weight – and your exercise efforts will be a waste of time.

A low calorie diet that's also low in saturated fat and unhealthy sugar, combined with regular exercise will go a long way to building a healthy physique. It sounds so easy, why then are many people unable to do it?

Most people do things on impulse. They see something on TV or hear a diet or workout that worked for a friend and they mimic it, without really understanding the why and the how. Diet and exercise should be tailored to your lifestyle. It should be something that you enjoy doing – to motivate you to keep on doing it. You need to have achievable and quantifiable targets so you can see the benefits of your efforts. Otherwise, if you're not happy about it, and you can't measure or see the results, you'll stop doing it at some point.

Dieting is hard to sustain. When we stop ourselves from eating a food we love, we feel deprived and this affects our overall mood and lowers our motivation. Understanding that you don't need to stop eating, but rather look for healthier counterparts, is the key.

There are low calorie versions of almost every food in the supermarket nowadays, choose those. Low cholesterol, no sugar, low fat – these are healthier options and they taste the same. Sugar is the hardest to remove from your diet, however, there are natural sweeteners available, such as Stevia. The secret is to educate yourself on the options available to you and know where to find them.

Here are delicious recipes that will assist in weight loss and remove belly fat, to make it easier for you to tone your abs. Try a combination of these suggested meals for 30 days and you will see visible results immediately. These are high fiber, low sugar, low fat and low calorie recipes. Healthy food doesn't have to be boring, just use the right ingredients.

The recommended daily allowance for the average man is 2500 and 2000 for the average woman. If you keep your daily calorie intake below these numbers, you will definitely lose weight.

# Breakfast Recipes

## Fruit and Vegetable Smoothies

When trying to lose weight, you can turn to healthy smoothies as a meal replacement. Choose ingredients that are packed with protein and high in fiber, to help keep you feeling full longer. Your imagination and creativity is the limit. Just avoid sugar and fruits that have large amounts of natural sugar such as mangoes.

Here's what you need to make a low calorie, healthy smoothie recipe for weight loss:

### Ingredients:

A Liquid Base (Non-fat milk, Greek Yogurt, Water)
Vegetables such as Spinach, Kale, Cabbage, Cauliflower
Fruits to mask the taste of the veggies (Banana, Apple, Avocado, Strawberries, Blueberries, Grapes)
Supplements (Optional - Fiber, Protein, etc.)
Stevia to sweeten
Ice

**Instructions:**

Put the liquid base in the blender and add the fruits. Blend.
While there are still chunks of fruit, add the vegetables.
Blend thoroughly.
Add Ice and Stevia, if you want it sweeter
Add supplements, if you need to.

Drink immediately.

# Oatmeal

Instead of cereal, try starting your day with a nice bowl of plain oats. Foods rich in protein keeps you going without getting hungry for a longer time.

If you put milk in your oatmeal, use Nonfat Milk and Stevia to sweeten.

# Egg White Muffin Cheese Melt

**Ingredients:**

3 Eggs, separate the white from the yolk
2 Whole Grain Egg Muffins or 2 Slices of Whole Wheat
bread
½ cup Spinach
1 slice low fat cheese
1 slice Tomato

**Instructions:**

Scramble the egg whites and cook lightly. Set aside.
Put the spinach on top of one egg muffin or 1 slice of
whole wheat bread
Put the cheese on the other bread
Toast the bread until the cheese melts
Add the egg and 1 slice tomato

# Apple Cinnamon Oats

## Ingredients:

Prepare 1 packet of plain instant oatmeal
½ cup skim milk
1small Apple, chopped
1 teaspoon cinnamon powder
Stevia to sweeten
Walnuts

## Instructions:

Cook the oatmeal and add the skim milk
Cook the apple, cinnamon and stevia mix in a microwave
Top the oatmeal with the apples.
Best eaten when hot.

# Strawberries and French Toast

## Ingredients:

2 slices whole wheat bread
1 egg
2 tbsp. skim milk
10 strawberries, sliced
Stevia to sweeten

## Instructions:

Beat the eggs and add the skim milk. Mix thoroughly
Dip the bread into the mixture
Cook in a non-stick pan until the bread is slightly browned
Top with the strawberries mixed with a little Stevia.

# Whole Wheat Pancakes and Berries

## Ingredients:

2 pcs. medium sized whole wheat pancakes
1 cup combination of blueberries and strawberries
1 tbsp. almond butter

## Instructions:

Spread the almond butter on the pancakes and top it off with ripe berries.

**Almond butter or almonds help keep your blood sugar levels steady. This will keep you **from craving for sweet foods.**

# Lunch Recipes

## Penne with Feta and Sun Dried Tomatoes

### Ingredients:

½ cup whole wheat pasta, cooked
1 cup spinach, sautéed
2 tbsp. pine nuts
2 tbsp. low fat feta
A handful of capers
Chopped sun-dried tomatoes

### Instructions:
Mix all ingredients together and spray some olive oil for texture and flavor

# Chopped Chicken Salad

## Ingredients:

3 ounces chopped chicken (roasted)
2 tbsps. crumbled blue cheese, low fat
½ cup cucumber, chopped
1 tbsp. chopped pecans
1 tbsp. dried cranberries
2 cup lettuce
2 tbsps. Vinaigrette

## Instructions:

Mix all ingredients together like a salad and top it off with the roasted chicken.

# Greek Quinoa and Avocados

## Ingredients:

½ cup uncooked Quinoa
2 plum tomatoes, seeds removed and chopped finely
2 avocados, pitted, sliced, meat only
1/3 cup grated feta cheese
1 cup water
½ cup shredded fresh spinach
1/3 cup finely chopped red onion
2 tbsps. Lemon juice
2 tbsps. Olive oil
½ tsp. salt
Spinach leaves

## Instructions:

Cook the quinoa like rice by combining it with the water in a saucepan.
In a bowl, combine the cooked quinoa with the tomatoes, onions and spinach
In a separate bowl, stir the lemon juice with the olive oil and add salt – mix it with the quinoa
Arrange the quinoa on a plate and add the spinach and avocado slices
Sprinkle the feta cheese on top.

# Black Bean Omelets

**Ingredients:**

1 can black beans, drained
Dash of hot sauce
1 Lime, juiced
4 eggs
4 egg whites
Salt and Pepper
½ avocado, sliced
4 tbsp. bottled salsa

**Instructions:**

Blend the black beans, hot sauce and lime in a food processor. Not too much.
Spray oil on a non-stick pan and heat over medium flame
Mix 1 egg, the egg whites, salt and pepper and whisk vigorously
Cook the eggs in a pan and lift the cooked egg with a spatula.
Arrange the egg in a plate.
On one side, spoon ¼ of the black bean mix and fold the egg into an omelet.
Top with avocado and salsa.

# Tuna Salad

## Ingredients:

3 oz. canned tuna, drained
1 tbsp. low fat mayonnaise
1 apple, diced
3 cups fresh spinach or kale
2 tbsps. Olive oil or vinegar dressing

## Instructions:

Combine the apple, mayo and tuna. Mix well. Serve over
the leafy greens and add the dressing.
Can be eaten cold.

# Dinner Recipes

## Chicken Corn Soup

### Ingredients:

4 oz. chicken breasts, strips
6 cups chicken stock
1 egg white
2 cups creamed corn
2 tsps. Salt
1 tsp. black pepper
1 tsp. sesame oil
¼ cup cornstarch
2 egg whites, beaten

### Instructions:

Cut the chicken into thin strips, or small cubes
Mix the chicken with 1 egg white and ½ cup of water
Heat chicken stock and add corn, salt, black pepper and sesame oil.
Add the marinated chicken to the stock.
Bring to a boil
Add the cornstarch mixed with ¼ cup of water
Add the beaten egg whites while mixing slowly and continuously. Serve hot!

# Baked Parmesan Fish

## Ingredients:

16 oz. fish fillet
2 tbsps. Milk
1 egg

Breading:
2 tbsps. Flour
1/3 cup grated parmesan cheese
¼ tsp. salt
½ tsp. paprika
1 pinch pepper

## Instructions:

In a sealable bag, combine breading ingredient. Set aside.
Beat the egg in a bowl and add milk
Dip the fillets in the batter one at a time
Shake off excess batter and then put the chicken fillet inside
the sealable bag and shake
Lay out the breaded fillets in an oiled sheet and bake at 350
degrees for 20 to 30 minutes
(once cooked, the fish will flake easily)
Serve with lemon if desired.

# Broccoli Casserole

## Ingredients:

3 boxes of frozen broccoli, chopped, thawed
1 can Cream of Mushroom
1 cup grated cheddar cheese
2 eggs, beaten
1 cup low fat mayonnaise
3 tbsps. Onions, grated
1 tbsp. white vinegar
unsalted crackers

## Instructions:

Mix all ingredients in a casserole dish
Crush the crackers and sprinkle on top
Bake the casserole for 45 minutes at 350 degrees.

# Healthy Fish Sticks

## Ingredients:

3 fillets of Tilapia (or your choice of fish)
1 ½ cups breadcrumbs
½ tsp. sea salt
2 egg whites, beaten
½ tsp pepper
¼ cup parmesan cheese

## Instructions:

Preheat the oven at 450 degrees
Lay a wire rack on top of a baking sheet and spray with non-stick
Cut the tilapia in bite sizes. Season with salt and pepper
In a bowl, beat the egg whites
In a separate bowl, mix the breadcrumbs, salt, pepper and cheese
Dip the fish sticks in the egg white, coating both sides
Then roll it in the breadcrumbs mixture, lightly pressing
Lay the fillets on the wire rack and spray with olive oil
Bake for 10 minutes. Then turn it over and bake for another 10.
Serve hot with low fat mayonnaise or catsup.

# Salmon with Cucumber Dill Sauce

## Ingredients:

1 cup water
1 lb. Salmon Fillet
1 cup dry white wine
1 tbsp. lemon juice
¾ non-fat yogurt
½ cup cucumber, unpeeled, finely chopped
¼ tsp. salt
1 tsp. dried dill

## Instructions:

Combine the white wine, water and lemon juice.
In a pan, bring the mixture to a boil, medium heat
Lower the heat and add the salmon
Simmer for 8 minutes or until the fish flakes easily
Combine the yogurt, cucumber, dill and salt. Stir thoroughly
Transfer the salmon to a plate, making sure it doesn't crumble. Use 2 spatulas.
Pour the cucumber sauce on the salmon
Add vegetables as a side dish

# The Belly Busters

Raw Almonds, Walnuts (All kinds of Nuts)
Greek Yogurt (Low Fat, Low Sugar)
Apples
Celery
Berries
Cucumber Sticks
Carrots
Unsweetened Oatmeal
Low calorie Smoothies
Flaxseeds
Natural Peanut Butter
Spicy Food
Bell Peppers
Beans
Olive Oil and Canola Oil
Whole grain and whole wheat breads and cereals
Protein Powder
Eggs
Low Fat Cheese
Lean Meat
Asparagus
Green Tea

# The Belly Builders

High Carbohydrate Foods
White Rice
Bread
Crackers
Bagels
Pasta
Cereals
Trans Fat
Omega-6 Fat and Saturated Fat
Packaged food
Processed Meat
Corn Oil
Soybean Oil
Milk and High Lactose
Dairy Food
High in Fructose
Sugar
Apples
Mangoes
Watermelon
Asparagus
Carbonated Drinks
High Sugar Drinks
Soda Drinks

# CONCLUSION

Over the years, a flat and toned midsection has been our benchmark for fitness. But a flat stomach means something else. It is the mark of people who are in control of their bodies, and therefore their health. We want to join that group.

For 30 days, do 30-minute exercises daily, mixing the exercises we showed you in the first chapters. Then, follow a high protein, low fat, low sugar and low calorie diet. You can try the recipes we suggested, or if you're a good cook, come up with a diet plan. Avoid the Belly Builders we mentioned to see the results of your efforts after 30 days.

There's hope of losing those jelly rolls and love handles yet. You just need to know what to do and how to do it – and stick to it.

We hope you found this book helpful and that after 30 days, you'll see less belly fat and more awesome abs like you've always wanted.

Thanks again for reading. Here's to a healthier you! Also, don't forget to grab our free weight loss report to maximize your chances of success at **flatbellyqueens.com**

Finally, if you enjoyed this book, then I'd like to ask you for a favor: would you be kind enough to leave a review for this book on Amazon? It'd be greatly appreciated!

Thank you and good luck!

# You may also like this book…

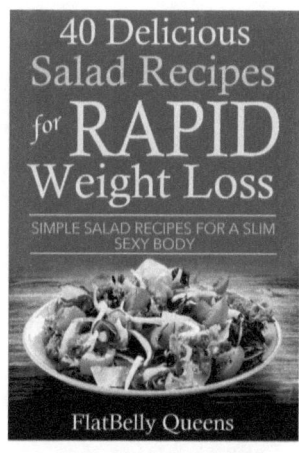

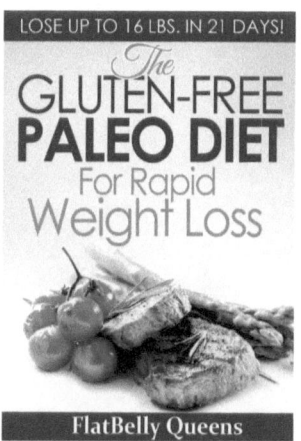

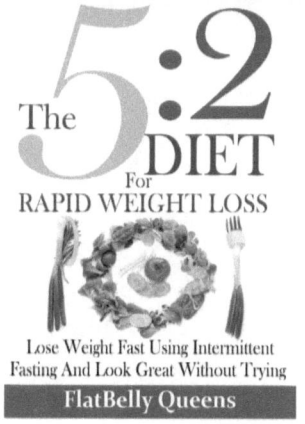

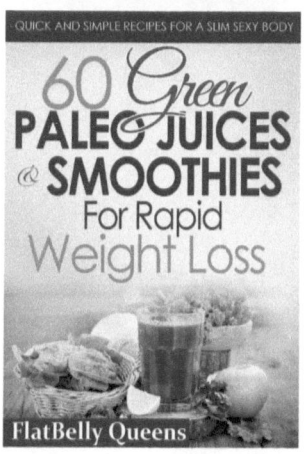